A Treatise on Bread

by

Sylvester Graham

HISTORY OF BREAD.

Primitive food of man. Bruising and grinding grain. Baking. Invention of leavened bread. Bread among the Greeks and Romans—among the Hebrews. Simplicity of the bread now used in many countries.

In the English version of the sacred scriptures, the term Bread is frequently used to signify vegetable food in general. Thus in Gen. iii, 19, the Lord says to Adam—"In the sweat of thy face shalt thou eat bread (or food) till thou return to the ground." See also Gen. xviii, 5, and xxviii, 20, and Ex. ii, 20.

The most extended sense of the word, however, according to general usage, comprehends all farinaceous vegetable substances which enter into the diet of man; such as the farinaceous seeds or grain, nuts, fruit, roots, &c. And in this extended sense, Bread, in some form or other, has been the principal article in the diet of mankind, from the earliest generations of the human race, to the present time; except among the few, small and scattered tribes, which have, perhaps, ever since the days of Noah, in different parts of the earth, subsisted mainly on animal food.

It is nearly certain that the primitive inhabitants of the earth, ate their food with very little, if any artificial preparation.

The various fruits, nuts, seeds, roots, and other vegetable substances on which they fed, were eaten by them in their natural state, with no other grinding than that which was done by the teeth.

As the human family increased, and population became more dense and extended, and providential measures more necessary, the condition and circumstances of society gradually led to the invention and adoption of the simple, and, at first, rude arts of domestic life. Among these, was that of bruising the harder articles of their food, such as nuts and seeds, or grain, on flat stones, selected and kept for the purpose. By constant use, these stones in time became hollowed out; and being thereby rendered more convenient, men at length began to form mortars and pestles from stones; and probably the next step was the construction of the rude kind of hand-mills, which continued in use for many centuries; and indeed, which, with the stone mortars, have, throughout all ages and in almost every portion of the earth, been used in the ruder states of society.

When men became acquainted with the use of fire, they probably often parched their corn or grain before they pounded it; and afterwards, they learned to mix it with water into the consistency of dough, and to bake this, in an unleavened or unfermented state, on flat stones before the fire, or in the hot ashes or hot earth, or in the rude ovens which they formed, by digging holes in the earth, into which they put heated stones, and slightly covered them with leaves or grass, and then laid in the article they wished to bake, and over this strewed some leaves, and then covered the whole with earth.[A]

This kind of unleavened bread, undoubtedly constituted a very important, if not the principal article of artificially prepared food in the diet of the primitive inhabitants of the earth, for many centuries; and the same, or very nearly the same kind of bread continued in general use down to the days of Abraham; and it is probable that the unleavened bread used by his descendants at the feast of the Passover, before and after they left Egypt, was of the same kind.

It is hardly possible, however, that it could have been otherwise, than that, at a much earlier period, larger quantities of this dough were occasionally made, than were immediately baked, and consequently portions of it were suffered to stand and ferment; and by this means, men were in process of time learned to make leavened, or raised bread.

At how early a date, loaf or raised bread came into common use, it is impossible now to ascertain with any considerable degree of precision. The scriptures do not afford us any evidence that Abraham was accustomed to such bread; but the fact that Moses, at the institution of the supper of the Passover, the night before the Jews left Egypt, commanded them strictly to abstain from leavened bread, and to eat only the unleavened, proves conclusively, that the Israelites at least, were then accustomed to fermented, or raised bread.

Neither history nor tradition enables us to speak with any degree of confidence in regard to the period at which other nations became acquainted with the art of bread-making; but from all that has come down to us from ancient times, we learn that the primitive generations of every nation, subsisted on fruits and other products of the vegetable kingdom, in their uncooked or natural state.

"The Greeks assert that they were taught the art of making bread by their god, Pan; and Pliny informs us that this art was not known at Rome till near six hundred years after the foundation of that city. The Roman armies, he says, on their return from Macedonia, brought Grecian bakers into Italy. Before this time, the Romans prepared their meal in a kind of pap or soft pudding; and on this account Pliny calls them pap eaters."

But though the Egyptians and Israelites were probably among the earliest portions of the human family, who became acquainted with the art of making loaf or raised bread, the quality of their bread continued to be exceedingly simple and coarse for many generations.

Even after the establishment of the Hebrew nation in Palestine—in the most splendid days of Jerusalem—at the period of the highest refinement of the Jews, in the arts of civil and domestic life, their fine flour, from which their choicest bread and cakes were made, was, in comparison with modern superfine flour, extremely coarse,—ground mostly by females, in hand-mills constructed and kept for that purpose.

From Rome the art of bread-making very slowly found its way over considerable portions of Europe. A thousand years after Julius Cæsar first entered Britain, the rude people of that country were little acquainted with raised bread. "Even at present," says Prof. Thomson, "loaf bread is seldom used except by the higher classes of inhabitants, in the northern countries of Europe and Asia."

In Eastern and Southern Asia, rice constitutes the principal bread-stuff; and this is generally prepared with great simplicity. In Middle and Western Asia, and in Africa, bread, though made of different kinds of grain, is prepared with almost equal simplicity. In Scotland, Ireland, and indeed throughout Europe generally, barley, oats, rye, potatoes, peas, beans, chesnuts, and other farinaceous vegetables, constitute the bread-stuff of most of the laboring people, or peasantry. In the islands of the Pacific and Southern oceans, the bread of the inhabitants consists of the plantain, bananas, yams, bread-fruit, and other like vegetables, simply roasted, baked, or boiled.

Bread, therefore, of some kind or other, made of some of the farinaceous products of the vegetable kingdom, has probably, in almost every portion of the world, and every period of time, been one of the first, and most important, and universal articles of food, artificially prepared by cooking, which has entered into the diet of mankind; and hence it has with great propriety been called "the staff of life."

LAWS OF DIET.

Reasons why food in its natural state would be the best. Concentrated nutriment. Interesting experiments on animals. Mixtures of food. Leavened and unleavened bread. Qualifications of the best bread.

If man were to subsist wholly on alimentary substances in their natural state, or without any artificial preparation by cooking, then he would be obliged to use his teeth freely in masticating his food; and by so doing, not only preserve his teeth from decay, and keep them in sound health, but at the same time, and by the same means, would he thoroughly mix his food with the fluid of his mouth, and thus prepare it both for swallowing and for the action of the stomach, and by the same means also, he would be made to swallow his food slowly, as the welfare of the stomach and of the whole system requires he should.

Again, if man were to subsist wholly on uncooked food, he would never suffer from the improper temperature of his aliment. Hot substances taken into the mouth, serve more directly and powerfully to destroy the teeth, than any other cause which acts immediately upon them; and hot food and drink received into the stomach, always in some degree debilitate that organ, and through it, every other organ and portion of the whole system; diminishing, as an ultimate result, the vital power of every part—impairing every function, and increasing the susceptibility of the whole body to the action of disturbing causes, and predisposing it to disease. Again, if man were to subsist entirely on food in a natural state, he would never suffer from concentrated aliment. Every substance in nature which God has prepared for the food of man, consists of both nutritious and innutritious matter. The proportions vary in different kinds of food. Thus in a hundred pounds of potatoes, there are about twenty-five pounds of nourishing matter; while in a hundred pounds of good wheat there are about eighty pounds of nourishing matter. There are a few products of the vegetable kingdom which are still higher in the scale of nutriment, than wheat; and on the other hand there is a boundless variety ranging below wheat, extending down to three or four per cent. of nourishment. But nature, without the aid of human art, produces nothing for the alimentary use of man which is purely a concentrated nutrient substance. And God has constructed man in strict accordance with this general economy of nature. He has organized and endowed the human body with reference to the condition and qualities of those substances in nature, which He designed for the food of man. And consequently, while man obeys the laws of constitution and relation which should govern him in regard to his food, he preserves the health and integrity of his alimentary organs, and through them of his whole nature; and so far as his dietetic habits are concerned, secures the highest and best condition of his nature. But, if he disregards these laws, and by artificial means greatly departs from the natural adaptation of things, he inevitably brings evil on himself and on his posterity.

It has been fully proved that "bulk, or a due proportion of innutritious matter in our food, is quite as important to health as nourishment." Human beings may subsist from childhood to extreme old age on good potatoes and pure water alone, and enjoy the best and most uninterrupted health, and possess the greatest muscular power and ability to endure protracted fatigue and exposure. But if the purely nutrient matter of the potato be separated out by artificial means, and human beings, fed exclusively on this concentrated form of aliment and pure water, they will soon perish, because the alimentary organs of man are not constituted and endowed for such kinds of food. And this is true of all animals, in the higher orders, at least.

We know that dogs fed on sugar and water, gum and water, fine flour bread and water, or any other kind of concentrated aliment, will soon languish, and droop, and emaciate, and die; but if a due proportion of proper innutritious substance be mixed with these concentrated forms of aliment, the dogs will subsist on them and remain healthy. So if horses, cows, deer, sheep, and other grass-eating animals be fed on grain alone, they will soon lose their appetite and begin to droop, and will shortly perish; but if a due proportion of straw or shavings of wood be given them with their grain, they will continue to do well. Man is affected in the same manner. He cannot long subsist on purely nutritious substances. And the reason is not because these substances have no azote or nitrogen in them; nor is it because man *necessarily* requires a variety of alimentary substances, but simply and exclusively because the anatomical construction and vital powers of the alimentary organs, are constitutionally adapted to alimentary substances which consist of both nutritious and innutritious matter; and therefore a due proportion of innutritious matter in the food of man is as essential to the welfare of his alimentary organs, as a due proportion of nourishment is to the support of his body.

Again, if man subsisted wholly on uncooked food, he would not only be preserved from improper concentrations, but also from pernicious combinations of alimentary substances. The alimentary organs of man, like those of the horse, ox, sheep, dog, cat, and most or all other animals of the higher orders, if not in fact, of all other animals without limitation, possess the vital capability of so accommodating themselves to emergencies, that they can be made to digest almost every vegetable and animal substance in nature; and they can, by long training, be educated to digest a mixture of these substances at the same time. Nevertheless it is incontestibly true, that the alimentary organs of man and of all other animals, can manage one kind of food at a time better than a mixed ingestion; for it is impossible that the solvent fluids secreted by the stomach and other organs belonging to the alimentary apparatus, should be at the same time equally well adapted to entirely different kinds of food.

I do not say that the alimentary organs of man cannot, by long habit, be brought into such a condition as that, while that condition remains, they will not manage a mixed ingestion of animal and vegetable food, with more immediate comfort and satisfaction to themselves and the individual, than they will an ingestion of pure vegetable food. But this does not militate against the general principle in the least; for it is nevertheless true, that the same organs are capable of being brought into a condition in which they will manage an ingestion of unmixed food of either kind, with less embarrassment and injury to themselves and the whole system, than they can the mixed food in any condition. Hence it is a general law of nature, concerning the dietetic habits of man, that simplicity of food at each meal is essential to the highest well-being of the individual and of the race.

God has unquestionably provided a great and rich variety of substances for man's nourishment and enjoyment; but it is equally certain that he did not design that man should partake of all this variety at a single meal, nor in a single day, nor season—but from meal to meal, from day to day, and from season to season, varying his enjoyment in strictest consistency with the great laws of his nature. And hence all artificial combinations of alimentary substances, and particularly those of a heterogeneous kind, and yet more especially the concentrated forms, must be more or less pernicious to the alimentary organs, and through them to the whole system.

Finally, if man subsisted wholly on uncooked food, the undepraved integrity of his appetite, his thorough mastication and slow swallowing, and his simple meal, would greatly serve to prevent his overeating, and thus save him from the ruinous effects of one of the most destructive causes operating in civic life.

Whatever may be the material, therefore, from which bread is made, when the artificial preparation is of that simple character which leaves the proportions of nutritious and innutritious properties, as nature combined them, and effects little change in the nutritious principles, and retains the natural requisition for the function of the teeth, and thus secures the proper chewing of the food and the mixing of it with the fluids of the mouth, and swallowing of it slowly, the artificial process militates very little, if at all, against any of the physiological or vital interests of the body. But if our artificial process of bread-making, concentrates the nutrient properties, and destroys the due proportion between the bulk and nourishment, and forms improper changes and combinations in the nutrient elements, and does away the necessity for mastication or chewing, and presents the food in too elevated a temperature, or too hot, and enables us to swallow it too rapidly, with little or no exercise of the teeth, and without properly mixing it with the fluids of the mouth, the artificial process or cooking is decidedly and often exceedingly inimical, not only to the vital interests of the alimentary organs, but of the whole human system.

In all civilized nations, and particularly in civic life, bread, as I have already stated, is far the most important article of food which is artificially prepared; and in our country and climate, it is the most important article that enters into the diet of man; and therefore it is of the first consideration, that its character should, in every respect, be as nearly as possible, consistent with the laws of constitution and relation established in our nature; or with the anatomical construction and vital properties and powers and interest of our systems.

If we contemplate the human constitution in its highest and best condition,—in the possession of its most vigorous and unimpaired powers —and ask, what must be the character of our bread in order to preserve that constitution in that condition? the answer most indubitably is, that the coarse unleavened bread of early times, when of proper age, was one of the least removes from the natural state of food,—one of the simplest and most wholesome forms of artificial preparations, and best adapted to fulfil the laws of constitution and relation; and therefore best adapted to sustain the most vigorous and healthy state of the alimentary organs, and the highest and best condition of the whole nature of man, as a general and permanent fact; and hence it is very questionable whether loaf or raised bread can be made equally conducive to all the interests of our nature, with the simple unleavened bread.

I am aware that many professional men entertain a very different opinion on this subject, and speak of unleavened bread as being less nourishing and less easily digested. This may be true to a limited extent, in special cases of impaired and debilitated alimentary organs; but I am confident that as a general fact the notion is entirely erroneous.

"The whole people of Asia," says Dr. Cullen, "live upon unfermented rice. The Americans, before they became acquainted with the Europeans, employed, and for the most part, still employ their maize in the same condition. Even in Europe, the employment of unfermented bread, and unfermented farinaceæ in other forms, is still very considerable, and we are ready to maintain that the morbid consequences of such a diet are very seldom to be observed. In Scotland, nine tenths of the lower classes of people—and that is the greater part of the whole—live upon unfermented bread and unfermented farinaceæ in other forms, and at the same time, I am of opinion that there are not a more healthy people anywhere to be found. We give it to all classes and both sexes with advantage."

It is incontestibly true, that if two portions of the same kind of wheat meal be taken and made, the one into unleavened and the other into leavened bread, and both be eaten warm from the oven, the leavened bread will prove much more oppressive and difficult to manage in the stomach than the unleavened. But aside from the changes that are produced by the process of fermentation, there are many other considerations why unleavened bread of a proper quality and age, is better adapted to sustain the alimentary organs and general constitution of man, in their highest and best condition.

Nevertheless, it is very certain, that loaf or raised bread can be made so nearly in accordance with the vital laws and interests of our bodies, as scarcely to militate against them in any perceptible or appreciable degree.

And when I say this, I mean not merely its effects on the health and longevity of a single individual, but its effects upon the human constitution, through successive generations, for a thousand years or more.

As a general criterion or rule, then, in regard to the character of bread, we perceive that the most perfect loaf or raised bread, is that which, being made of the best material, is light, and sweet, and well baked, and still most nearly retains all the natural proportions and properties of the original material.

MATERIAL OF BREAD.

Wheat. Extent of climate favorable to it. Injured by improper tillage. Removal of impurities. Washing of grain. Separation of the bran from the nutrient particles improper. Ancient Roman bread. Public bakers. Use of bad flour. Adulterations. Poisonous agents used to disguise them.

Among the materials used for making bread in our country—and, in fact, of all the known productions of the vegetable kingdom in any country, wheat is decidedly the best; and it is a remarkable fact, that wheat comes nearer to man than perhaps any other plant, in its power of becoming adapted to different climates, over a wide extent of the earth's surface, so that it may almost be said that wherever the human species can flourish, there wheat can be cultivated.

"It is not certainly known," says Prof. Thomson, "in what country wheat was first produced. Mr. Bruce informs us that he found it growing wild in Abyssinia; and in his opinion, that kingdom is the native country of the plant. It would seem," continues the Professor, "to be originally an African plant, since it thrives best in Barbary and Egypt; and perhaps the mountains of Abyssinia, though within the torrid zone, may not differ much in point of climate, from the more northern plains of Egypt. Wheat is perhaps cultivated over a greater extent of the globe than any other plant. Excellent crops are raised as far north as Sweden, in latitude 60°; it is cultivated in the East Indies, considerably within the limits of the torrid zone; and in the North of Hindostan, it constitutes a chief article in the food of the inhabitants. In India, however, the plant seems to have deteriorated. It is always dwarfish, and the crop is said to be less abundant than in more northern climates." Yet a cold climate is not most genial to the nature of this plant. "The wheat of France is superior to that of England; the wheat of

Italy is still better than that of France; and perhaps the best of all is raised in Barbary and Egypt."

Excellent wheat is raised in the southern, and western, and middle portions of the United States; and even in the northern and eastern parts of New England, very fine crops have been produced.

But the wheat and other cultivated products of the vegetable kingdom appropriated to the nourishment of man, like those on which our domestic animals subsist, are too generally, in civilized life, very considerably deteriorated, as to their wholesomeness, by the improper tillage of the soil. I have no doubt that it is true, as stated by those who have made the experiment, that the flour of wheat, raised on a cultivated soil recently dressed with crude, stable manure, may readily be distinguished by its odor, from the flour of wheat raised on a new and undepraved soil, or from that raised on a cultivated soil which has been dressed with properly digested manure. And if such and similar results of improper tillage can become the sources of serious evil to the human family, through their effects on the flesh of animals which man devours, and on the milk and butter which he consumes, surely the immediate effects of such a deteriorated vegetable aliment on the human system, must be very considerable.

They who have never eaten bread made of wheat, recently produced by a pure virgin soil, have but a very imperfect notion of the deliciousness of good bread; such as is often to be met with in the comfortable log houses in our western country. It is probably true that the new soil, in its virgin purity, before it becomes exhausted by tillage, and debauched by the means which man uses to enrich and stimulate it, produces most, if not all kinds of vegetables appropriate for human aliment, in a more perfect and healthy state, than any soil which has been long under cultivation, can be made to do. Nevertheless, by a proper application of physiological principles to agriculture, many of the evils which now result from improper tillage may easily be avoided, and the quality of all those vegetable substances which enter into the diet of man may be very greatly improved, both in regard to wholesomeness and deliciousness.

But while the people of our country are so entirely given up as they are at present, to gross and promiscuous feeding on the dead carcasses of animals, and to the untiring pursuits of wealth, it is perhaps wholly in vain for a single individual to raise his voice on a subject of this kind. The farmer will continue to be most eager to increase the number of his acres, and to extort from those acres the greatest amount of produce, with the least expense of tillage, and with little or no regard to the quality of that produce in relation to the physiological interests of man; while the people generally, are contented to gratify their depraved appetites on whatever comes before them, without pausing to inquire whether their indulgences are adapted to preserve or to destroy their health and life. Yet if some one does not raise a voice upon this subject which shall be heard and heeded, there will soon reach us, as a nation, a voice of calamity which we shall not be able to shut our ears against, albeit we may in the perverseness of our sensualism, incorrigibly persist in disregarding its admonitions, till the deep chastisements of outraged nature shall reach the very "bone and marrow" of the human constitution, and fill our land with such a living rottenness, as now in some other portions of the earth, renders human society odious and abominable.

Whether, therefore, my voice shall be heard and heeded or not, I will obey the dictates of my sense of duty, and solemnly declare that this subject demands the prompt and earnest attention of every agriculturist and of every friend to the common cause of humanity; for it is most certain, that until the agriculture of our country is conducted in strict accordance with physiological truth, it is not possible for us to realize those physical, and intellectual, and moral, and social, and civil blessings for which the human constitution and our soil and climate are naturally capacitated.

When proper attention has been paid to the character of the wheat itself, the next thing is to see that it is thoroughly cleansed.

Sometimes, in consequence of the peculiarities of the season, or climate, or soil, or some other cause, there will be a species of disease affecting the wheat and other grains; and this may be of such a character as not easily to be removed nor counteracted by any means; but more generally the rust, and smut, and dust, which attach themselves to the skin of the grain, may, by proper care, be so far removed, as at least to render the meal or flour far more pure and wholesome than it otherwise would be. And here let me remark, that they are greatly deceived, who suppose that the bolting cloth which separates the fine flour from the outer skin or bran, also separates the impurities attached to the outer skin from the flour. By the process of grinding, these impurities are rubbed from the outer skin, and made quite as fine as any portion of the flour, and for the most part pass with the fine flour through the bolting cloth.

To remedy this, it is perhaps generally true, that in large flouring establishments, a kind of smut or scouring mill is in operation, through which the wheat passes, and is pretty thoroughly rubbed or scoured without being broken; and after this, it passes through a screen or winnowing mill, and thus is tolerably well cleansed and prepared for grinding. Yet this process by no means renders the wheat so perfectly clean and wholesome as washing.

Those who have given little attention to this subject, will probably think that the trouble of washing all their bread-stuff before it is ground, would be much greater than any benefit which would result from it. But a short experience in the matter, would convince every one who has a proper regard for the character of his bread, that the trouble of washing his grain bears no comparison to the improvement effected by it. Indeed, they who become accustomed to washing their grain, will soon cease to regard it as a trouble;

and the improvement in the whiteness and sweetness of their bread will be so great, that they would be extremely unwilling to relinquish the practice.

When people are so situated that they can have things as they wish, they will also find that their bread is much richer, if the grain is ground but a short time before it is cooked.

The best way, therefore, is, for every family to raise or purchase a sufficient quantity of the best new wheat that can be produced by proper tillage in a good soil, and put that away in clean casks or bins, where it will be kept perfectly dry and sweet; and, according to the size of the family, take, from time to time, as they need it, one or two bushels, and wash it thoroughly but briskly in two or three waters, and then spread it out on a drying sheet or table, made for the purpose, and which is considerably inclined, so that the water remaining with the wheat will easily run off.

The skin or bran of the wheat is so well protected by its own oily property, that little or no water will penetrate it, unless it be suffered to remain in the water much longer than is necessary. Being thinly spread out upon the sheet or table in a good drying day, it will be sufficiently dry in a few hours for grinding. And I say again, let any one who loves good bread, wash his grain a few times in this manner, and he will be very reluctant to return to the use of bread made of unwashed grain.

It would be difficult to ascertain at how early a period in the progress of society, mankind, in the preparation of wheat for bread-making, began to put asunder what God has joined together, and to concentrate the more purely nutrient properties, by separating the flour from the part commonly called the bran. The Bible speaks of fine flour or meal, as a portion of the meat offerings of the temple, but it is not probable this approached very near to the superfine flour of the present time.

We are informed also that the Romans, more than two thousand years ago, had four or five different kinds of bread—one of which was made of the purest flour, from which all the bran was separated. This was eaten only by the rich and luxurious. A second kind, in more common use, was that from which a portion of the bran was taken; and a third kind, which was more generally used than any other, was that which was made of the whole substance of the wheat. A fourth kind was made mostly of the bran, for dogs.

But at whatever period in the history of the race, this artificial process was commenced, certain it is that in direct violation of the laws of constitution and relation which the Creator has established in the nature of man, this process of mechanical analysis is, at the present day, carried to the full extent of possibility; and the farina, and gluten, and saccharine matter of the wheat, are almost perfectly concentrated in the form of superfine flour. Nor is this all—these concentrated nutrient properties of the wheat are mixed and complicated in ways innumerable, with other concentrated substances, to pamper the depraved appetites of man, with kinds of food which always and inevitably tend to impair his health and to abbreviate his life.

Even the bread, which is the simplest form into which human ingenuity tortures the flour of wheat, is, by other causes besides the concentration I have named, too frequently rendered the instrument of disease and death, rather than the means of life and health, to those that eat it.

In cities and large towns, most people depend on public bakers for their bread. And I have no doubt that public bakers, as a body, are as honest and worthy a class of men as any in society. I have no wish to speak evil of any one; and it is always painful to me to find myself compelled, in fidelity to the common cause of humanity, to expose the faults of any particular class of men, when probably every other class in society is as deeply involved in errors which, in the sight of God, evince, at least, an equal degree of moral turpitude.

But public bakers, like other men, who serve the public more for the sake of securing their own emolument than for the public good, have always had recourse to various expedients in order to increase the lucrativeness of their business.

To secure custom and profit at the same time, they have considered it necessary, that a given quantity of flour should be made into a loaf as large and as white as possible, and free from any disagreeable taste, while at the same time it retains the greatest possible weight.

From a variety of causes, the quality and price of flour have always been very unstable. Sometimes the crops are small, or the foreign demand for flour or the home consumption is unusually great, or the season is unfavorable to the health of grain, and the wheat becomes diseased, or the harvest time is unfavorable, and the wheat sprouts before it is secured, or large quantities of flour become soured or musty, or in some other manner damaged.

To counteract these things, and to make the most profitable use of such flour as the market affords them, the public bakers have been led to try various experiments with chemical agents, and there is reason to believe that in numerous instances, they have been too successful in their practices, for the well-being of those who have been the consumers of their bread.

According to treatises on bread-making, which have within a few years past appeared in European scientific journals, "alum, sulphate of zinc, sub-carbonate of magnesia, sub-carbonate of ammonia, sulphate of copper, and several other substances, have been used by public bakers in making bread; and some of these substances have been employed by them to a very great extent, and with very great success in the cause of their cupidity. They have not only succeeded by such means, in making light and white bread out of extremely poor flour, but they have also been able so to disguise their adulterations, as to work in with their flour, without being detected by the consumers, a portion of the flour of beans, peas and potatoes—and even chalk, pipe clay and plaster of Paris, have been employed to increase the weight and whiteness of their bread."

"The use of alum in bread-making," says a distinguished chemist, "appears to be very ancient. It is one of those articles which have been the most extensively and successfully used in disguising bad flour, and the various adulterations of bread. Its injurious action upon the health is not to be compared with that of sulphate of copper, and yet, daily taken into the stomach, it may seriously affect the system."

"Thirteen bakers were condemned on the 27th of January, 1829, by the correctional tribunal of Brussels, for mixing sulphate of copper or blue vitriol with their bread. It makes the bread very white, light, large and porous, but rather tasteless; and it also enables the bread to retain a greater quantity of water, and thereby very considerably increases its weight. A much larger quantity of alum is necessary to produce these effects; but when of sufficient quantity, it strengthens the paste, and, as the bakers say, 'makes the bread swell large.'"

If the statements of our large druggists can be relied on, the public bakers of our own country probably employ ammonia more freely, at present, than any other substance I have named. Pearlash or saleratus is also used by them in considerable quantities.

But even where these adulterations are not practised, the bakers' bread is very rarely a wholesome article of diet.

If any dependence is to be placed on the testimony of several of the principal bakers and flour merchants in New York, Boston and other cities, the flour which most of our public bakers work into bread, is of a very inferior quality to what is called good "family flour," and for which they pay from one to three dollars less per barrel; and they sometimes purchase large quantities of old spoiled flour from New Orleans and elsewhere, which has heated and soured in the barrel, and perhaps become almost as solid as a mass of chalk; so that they are obliged to break it up, and grind it over, and spread it out, and expose it to the air, in order to purify it in a measure from its acid and other bad properties; and then they mix it with a portion of much better flour; and from this mixture they can make, as they say, the very largest and finest looking loaf.[B]

But should the public bakers always use the best of flour, their bread, as a general statement, would still be very inferior to well made domestic bread, in point of sweetness and wholesomeness. Their mode of manufacturing bread—to say the least of it—destroys much of the virtue of the flour or meal; and hence their bread is only palatable—even to those who are accustomed to it—within twelve, or at the longest, twenty-four hours after it is baked.

But I must repeat, that in making these statements, I am not prompted by any unkind feelings towards public bakers; I have no doubt that they are as honest in their calling as any other class of men; but perhaps there is no other class pursuing an interest founded on the necessities of their fellow creatures, whose expedients to increase the lucrativeness of their business, are so immediately and universally injurious to the health of those on whom they depend for support.

If any of my statements are thought to be exaggerated or incorrect, I can only say, that with honest and benevolent intentions, I have diligently sought for the truth; and if I have been in any respect betrayed into error, I have been misinformed by public bakers themselves, who certainly ought to know the truth in this matter; and who could have no conceivable reason for making the general character of their calling appear worse than it really is. Nevertheless, I have no question that there are individuals in every city employed as public bakers, who are too honest—too conscientious—too upright in heart, to be guilty of any practice which they consider fraudulent or improper.

Still, truth compels me to declare, that if we would have good and wholesome bread, it must be made within the precincts of our own domestic threshold; and by those whose skill and care are exercised more with a view to secure our health and happiness, than their own pecuniary interest.

PROPERTIES OF BREAD.

Superfine flour injurious—a probable cause of some common disorders. Objections to coarse bread. Its medical properties. Extensive experiments of its use, by soldiers and others. Use among European peasantry. Selection, preservation and grinding of wheat.

Whether our bread is of domestic manufacture or made by the public baker, that which is made of superfine flour is always far less wholesome, in any and every situation of life, than that which is made of wheaten meal which contains all the natural properties of the grain.

It is true, that when much flesh is eaten with our bread, or when bread constitutes but a very small and unimportant portion of our food, the injurious effects of superfine flour bread are not always so immediately and distinctly perceived as in other cases. Nevertheless, it is a general and invariable law of our nature, that all concentrated forms of food are unfriendly to the physiological or vital interests of our bodies.

A very large proportion of all the diseases and ailments in civic life, are originated by causes which are introduced into the alimentary canal as articles of diet; and disturbance and derangement of function—obstructions, debility and irritations, are among the most important elements of those diseases.

It is, probably, speaking within bounds, to say that nine tenths of the adults, and nearly as large a proportion of youth in civic life, are more or less afflicted with obstructions and disturbances in the stomach and bowels, and other organs of the abdomen, the symptoms of which are either habitual costiveness or diarrhœa, or an alternation of both; or frequent and severe attacks of what are called bilious colics, &c., &c.; and in children and youth, worms, fits, convulsions, &c. And I cannot but feel confident, that the use of superfine flour bread is among the important causes of these and numerous other difficulties.

I have indeed been surprised to observe, that in the hundreds of cases of chronic diseases of every form and name, which have come to my knowledge within the last five or six years, costiveness of the bowels has in almost every instance been among the first and most important symptoms. And I have never known this difficulty, even after an obstinate continuance of five, ten, twenty or thirty years, fail to disappear in a short time, after the coarse wheaten bread of a proper character has been substituted for that made of superfine flour.

Some physicians and other individuals, without properly examining the subject, have raised several objections against the coarse wheaten bread.

It is said, in the first place, that bran is wholly indigestible, and therefore should never be taken into the human stomach.

This objection betrays so much ignorance of the final causes and constitutional laws, clearly indicated by the anatomical structure and physiological economy of the alimentary organs, that it scarcely deserves the slightest notice. If the digestive organs of man were designed to receive nothing but digestible and nutrient substances, they would have been constructed and arranged very differently from what they are. As we have already seen, everything which nature provides for our sustenance, consists of certain proportions of nutritious and innutritious matter; and a due proportion of innutritious matter in our food is as essential to the health and functional integrity of our alimentary organs, as a due proportion of nutritious matter is to the sustenance of the body.

Another objection is, that although bran may serve, like other mechanical irritants and excitants, for a while, to relieve constipation, yet it soon wears out the excitability of the organs, and leaves them more inactive than before.

Here again, a false statement is urged by inexcusable ignorance; for it is not true that the bran acts in the manner supposed in this objection; nor are the effects here asserted ever produced by it.

It is true, however, that the very pernicious habits of some people, who use the coarse wheaten bread, entirely counteract the aperient effects of the bread; and it is true that others, depending wholly on the virtues of this bread for peristaltic action, and neglecting all exercise, by their extreme inertness, and indolence, and overeating, bring on a sluggishness, and debility, and constipation of the bowels, and perhaps become severely afflicted with piles, in spite of the natural fitness of the bread to promote regular peristaltic action, and to prevent all these results.

A third objection is, that though the coarse wheaten bread may do very well for those who are troubled with constipation, by mechanically irritating and exciting the stomach and bowels, yet for that very reason it is wholly unfit and improper for those who are afflicted with chronic diarrhœa.

Here is still another objection founded in ignorance of the true physiological and pathological principles which it involves. The truth is, that the coarse wheaten bread, under a proper general regimen, is as excellent and sure a remedy for chronic diarrhœa as for chronic constipation.

I have seen cases of chronic diarrhœa of the most obstinate character, and which had baffled the highest medical skill and every mode of treatment for more than twenty years, yielding entirely under a proper general regimen, in which this bread was the almost exclusive article of food, and not a particle of medicine was used. And I have never known such a mode of treatment to fail of wholly relieving diarrhœa, whether recent or chronic; although a very great number of cases have come under my notice.

It is fully evident, therefore, that the bran does not act on the digestive organs as a mere mechanical irritant; for if it did, it would always necessarily aggravate, rather than alleviate diarrhœa. Nor does it relieve diarrhœa on the principle of a narcotic nor of a stimulant; for the effect of these is always to give an immediate check to that complaint; and in such a manner as to expose the system to a return of it. But the coarse wheaten bread *seems* to increase the disease for a short time, at first, and then gradually restores the healthy condition and action of the bowels.

The mucilage of wheat bran is probably one of the most soothing substances in the vegetable kingdom, that can be applied to the mucous membrane of the stomach and bowels.

Chronic constipation and chronic diarrhœa, both spring from the same root. Where the constitutional vigor of the alimentary canal is very considerable, continued irritations, resulting in debility, will produce constipation; and these continued causes operating for some time, will often induce such a state of debility and irritability as is attended with diarrhœa: —and in other cases, when this constitutional vigor of the alimentary canal is much less, diarrhœa is far more readily induced, and rendered chronic.

Coarse wheaten bread, then, by its adaptation to the anatomical structure and to the physiological properties and functional powers of our organs, serves to prevent and to remove the disorders and diseases of our bodies, only by preventing and removing irritation and morbid action and condition, and thereby affording the system an opportunity of recovering its healthy and vigorous action and condition. And the thousands of individuals in our own country of every age—of both sexes—of all situations, conditions and circumstances, who within the last six years have been benefited by using the coarse wheaten bread, instead of that made of superfine flour, are living witnesses of the virtues of that bread.

But the testimony in favor of coarse wheaten bread as an important article in the food of man, is by no means limited to our own country nor to modern times.

In all probability, as we have already seen, the first generations of our species, who became acquainted with the art of making bread, continued for many centuries to employ all the substance of the grain, which they coarsely mashed in their rude mortars or mills. And even since mankind began, by artificial means, to separate the bran from the flour, and to make bread from the latter, the more close and discerning observers among physicians and philanthropists, have perceived and asserted, that bread made of fine flour is decidedly less wholesome than that made of the unbolted wheat meal.

Hippocrates, styled the father of medicine, who flourished more than two thousand years ago, and who depended far more on a correct diet and general regimen, both for the prevention and removal of disease, than he did on medicine, particularly commended the unbolted wheat meal bread, "for its salutary effects upon the bowels." It was a fact well understood by the ancients, that this bread was much more conducive to the general health and vigor of their bodies, and every way better adapted to nourish and sustain them than that made of the fine flour. And accordingly, their wrestlers and others who were trained for great bodily power, "ate only the coarse wheaten bread, to preserve them in their strength of limbs." The Spartans were famous for this kind of bread; and we learn from Pliny that the Romans, as a nation, at that period of their history when they were the most remarkable for bodily vigor and personal prowess and achievement, knew no other bread for three hundred years. The warlike and powerful nations which overran the Roman Empire, and finally spread over the greater part of Europe, used no other kind of bread than that which was made of the whole substance of the grain; and from the fall of the Roman Empire to the present day, a large proportion of the inhabitants of all Europe and the greater part of Asia, have rarely used any other kind of bread.

"If you set any value on health, and have a mind to preserve nature,"—said Thomas Tryon, student in physic, in his "Way to Health, Long Life and

Happiness," published in London, in the latter part of the fifteenth century,—"you must not separate the finest from the coarsest flour; because that which is fine is naturally of an obstructive and stopping quality; but, on the contrary, the other, which is coarse, is of a cleansing and opening nature, therefore the bread is best which is made of both together. It is more wholesome, easier of digestion, and more strengthening than bread made of the finest flour. It must be confessed, that the nutrimentive quality is contained in the fine flour; yet, in the branny part is contained the opening and digestive quality; and there is as great a necessity for the one as the other, for the support of health: that which is accounted the worst is as good and beneficial to nature as the best; for when the finest flour is separated from the coarsest and branny parts, neither the one nor the other has the true operations of the wheat meal. The eating of fine bread, therefore, is inimical to health, and contrary both to nature and reason; and was at first invented to gratify *wanton* and *luxurious* persons, who are ignorant both of themselves, and the true virtue and efficacy of natural things."

"Baron Steuben has often told me," says Judge Peters, "that the peculiar healthfulness of the Prussian soldiers, was in a great measure to be attributed to their ammunition bread, made of grain, triturated or ground, but not bolted; which was accounted the most wholesome and nutritious part of their rations."[C]

"The Dutch sailors, in the days of their naval glory, were supplied with the same kind of bread."

"During the war between England and France, near the close of the last century," says Mr. Samuel Prior, a respectable merchant of Salem, New Jersey—"the crops of grain, and particularly wheat, were very small in England, and the supplies from Dantzic, the Netherlands and Sweden being cut off by the French army, and also the usual supplies from America failing, there was a very great scarcity of wheat in England. The British army was then very extensive, and it was exceedingly difficult to procure provisions for it, both at home and abroad—on land and sea. Such was the demand for the foreign army, and such the deficiency of crops at home and supplies from abroad, that serious fears were entertained that the army would suffer, and that the continental enterprise of the British government would be defeated in consequence of the scarcity of provisions; and every prudential measure by which such a disastrous event could be prevented, was carefully considered and proposed. William Pitt was then prime minister of state, and at his instance, government recommended to the people generally throughout Great Britain, to substitute potatoes and rice as far as possible, for bread, in order to save the wheat for the foreign army. This recommendation was promptly complied with by many of the people. But still the scarcity was alarmingly great. In this emergency, parliament passed a law (to take effect for two years) that the army at home should be supplied with bread made of unbolted wheat meal, solely for the purpose of making the wheat go as far as possible, and thus saving as much as they could from the home consumption, for the better supply of the army on the continent.

"Eighty thousand men were quartered in barracks in the counties of Essex and Suffolk. A great many were also quartered throughout the towns, at taverns, in squads of thirty or forty in a place. Throughout the whole of Great Britain, the soldiers were supplied with this coarse bread. It was deposited in the store-rooms with the other provisions of the army; and on the day that it was baked, and at nine o'clock the next morning, was distributed to the soldiers—who were at first exceedingly displeased with the bread, and refused to eat it, often casting it from them with great rage, and violent execrations. But after two or three weeks they began to be much pleased with it, and preferred it to the fine flour bread.

"My father," continues Mr. P., "whom I have often heard talk these things over, was a miller and a baker, and resided in the county of Essex, on the border joining Suffolk, and near the barracks containing the eighty thousand soldiers. He contracted with government, to supply the eastern district of the county of Essex, with the kind of bread I have mentioned: and he used always to send me with it to the depositories on the day it was baked: and though I was then a youth, I can still very distinctly remember the angry looks and remarks of the soldiers, when they were first supplied with it. Indeed they often threw their loaves at me as I passed along, and accompanied them with a volley of curses. The result of this experiment was, that not only the wheat was made to go much farther, but the health of the soldiers improved so much and so manifestly, in the course of a few months, that it became a matter of common remark among themselves, and of observation and surprise among the officers and physicians of the army. These gentlemen at length came out with confidence and zeal on the subject, and publicly declared that the soldiers were never before so healthy and robust; and that disease of every kind had almost entirely disappeared from the army. The public papers, were for months filled with recommendations of this bread, and the civic physicians almost universally throughout Great Britain, pronounced it far the most healthy bread that could be eaten, and as such, recommended it to all the people, who very extensively followed the advice:—and the coarse wheaten bread was very generally introduced into families—female boarding schools, and indeed all public institutions. The nobility also generally used it; and in fact, in many towns, it was a rare thing to meet with a piece of fine flour bread. The physicians generally asserted that this wheaten bread was the very best thing that could be taken into the human stomach, to promote digestion and peristaltic action; and that it, more than anything else, would assist the stomach in digesting other things which were less easily digested, and therefore they recommend that a portion of it should be eaten at every meal with other food.

"Still, after this extensive experiment had been made with such happy results, and after so general and full a testimony had been given in favor of the coarse wheaten bread, when large supplies of superfine flour came in from America, and the crops at home were abundant, and the act of parliament in relation to the army became extinct, most of the people who had before been accustomed to the use of fine flour bread, now by degrees returned again to their old habits of eating fine bread. Many of the nobility, however, continued to use the coarse bread for a number of years afterwards. General Hanoward, Squire Western, Squire Hanbury and others living near my father's, continued to use the bread for a long time, and some of them still used it when I left home and came to America, in 1816."

The testimony of sea captains and old whalemen is equally in favor of wheaten bread. "I have always found," said a very intelligent sea captain of more than thirty years' experience, "that the coarser my ship bread, the healthier my crew is."

A writer in Rees' Cyclopædia, (article Bread) says—"The inhabitants of Westphalia, who are a hardy and robust people, and capable of enduring the greatest fatigues, are a living testimony to the salutary effects of this sort of bread; and it is remarkable that they are very seldom attacked by acute fevers, and those other diseases which are from bad humors."

In short, as I have already stated, the bread of a large portion of the laboring class, or peasantry, throughout Europe, Asia and Africa, and the islands of the ocean, whether leavened or unleavened—whether more or less artificially prepared, is made of the whole substance of the grain from which it is manufactured: and no one who is sufficiently enlightened in physiological science to qualify him to judge correctly in this matter, can doubt that bread made in the best manner from unbolted wheat meal, is far better adapted to the anatomical structure and physiological powers of the alimentary organs of man, than bread made of superfine wheat flour; and consequently, the former is far more conducive to the health and vigor and general well-being of man than the latter.

If, therefore, mankind will have raised bread which in every respect most perfectly conforms to the laws of constitution and relation established in their nature, and is most highly conducive to the welfare of their bodies and souls, then must it be well made, well baked, light and sweet bread, which contains all the natural properties of the wheat. And if they will have this bread of the very best, and most wholesome kind, they must, as I have already stated, see that the soil from which their wheat is raised, is of a proper character, and is properly tilled,—that the wheat is plump—full-grown—ripe, and free from rust and other diseases; and then, before it is ground, they must see that it is thoroughly cleansed, not only from chaff, cockles, tares, and such like substances, but also from all smut, and every kind of impurity that may be attached to the skin of the kernel. And let every one be assured that this is a matter which really deserves all the attention and care that I suggest.

If human existence is worth possessing, it is worth preserving; and they who have enjoyed it as some have done, and as all the human family are naturally endowed with the capabilities to enjoy it, certainly will not doubt whether it is worth possessing; nor, if they will properly consider the matter, can they doubt that its preservation is worthy of their most serious and diligent care.

And when they perceive how intimately and closely the character of their bread is connected with the dearest interests of man, they will not be inclined to feel that any reasonable amount of care and labor is too much to be given to secure precisely the right kind of bread.

I repeat, then, that they who would have the very best bread should certainly wash their wheat, and cleanse it thoroughly from all impurities, before they take it to the mill; and when it is properly dried, it should be ground by sharp stones which will cut rather than mash it: and particular care should be taken that it is not ground too fine. Coarsely ground wheat meal, even when the bran is retained, makes decidedly sweeter and more wholesome bread than very finely ground meal. When the meal is ground, it should immediately be spread out to cool before it is put into sacks or casks:—for if it is packed or enclosed in a heated state, it will be far more likely to become sour and musty. And I say again, where families are in circumstances to do wholly as they choose in the matter, it is best to have but little ground at a time; as the freshly ground meal is always the liveliest and sweetest, and makes the most delicious bread.

When the meal is thus prepared and brought home, whether in a barrel or sack, the next thing to be attended to, is, that it be placed and kept in a perfectly clean, and sweet, and well ventilated meal room. It should on no consideration be put into a closet, or pantry, or store-room, which is seldom aired, and more rarely cleansed; and into which all manner of rubbish is thrown; or even where other kinds of provisions are kept. If the meal be put into a pantry or store-room which is confined and dirty, and into which old boots and shoes, and old clothes and pieces of carpet, and other things of this kind, are thrown—or where portions of vegetable or animal substance, whether cooked or uncooked, are habitually or even occasionally put and permitted to remain, it must be expected, as a matter of course, of necessity, that the quality of the meal will be considerably deteriorated by the impurities with which the air of the place will be loaded, and which will be continually generated there.

People generally have but a sorry idea of what constitutes true cleanliness; but they may be assured that they cannot be too deeply impressed with the importance of keeping their meal room as clean and sweet and well aired as possible.

FERMENTATION.

Chemical composition of flour. Yeast—modes of preparing it. Substitutes for it. Fermentation, and its products. Vinous, acetous and putrefactive fermentation.

Having procured good wheat, cleansed it thoroughly, and got it properly ground, and placed in the meal room, the next step is to take a portion of the meal and manufacture it into good bread. But in order that this may be done in the most certain and perfect manner, it is important that the properties of the meal and the principles concerned in bread-making should be well understood.

According to the statement of Prof. Thomson, of Edinburgh, one pound of good wheat meal contains ten ounces of farina or starch, three ounces of bran, six drams of gluten and two drams of sugar;—and it is because wheat contains such proportions of these substances that it makes the very best loaf bread. The farina or starch is the principal nourishing property;—the saccharine matter or sugar is also highly nutrient; but in the process of making loaf bread, it serves mainly, by its vinous fermentation, to produce the gas or air by which the dough is raised and the bread made light. The gluten is likewise a very nutrient property, but in loaf bread, it principally serves, by its cohesiveness, like gum elastic, or India rubber, to prevent the gas or air formed by the fermentation of the sugar, from escaping or passing off;—and the gas being thus retained, inflates or puffs up the dough, and makes it porous and light. The bran, with its mucilaginous and other properties, not only adds to the nutritiousness of the bread, but eminently serves to increase its digestibility, and to invigorate the digestive organs, and preserve the general integrity of their functions.

The wheat which is raised in Virginia and the southern states generally, contains a larger proportion of gluten than that which is raised in the western part of the state of New York. Hence bakers are able to make a larger loaf of bread out of a pound of southern flour than they can out of a pound of western flour; and consequently some of them have endeavored to make their customers believe that the southern flour is the most profitable. It certainly *is* the most profitable for the baker; but it is not the most profitable for the consumer.

The next thing indispensably necessary to the making of good bread, is good lively sweet yeast, or leaven, to produce what is called the panary, or more properly, the vinous fermentation of the saccharine matter, or sugar.

Some bread-makers will do best with one kind of yeast or leaven, and some with another. I have generally found that people do best with those materials to which they have been most accustomed; but I am sorry to find so general a dependence on breweries for yeast. To say nothing of the impure and poisonous substances which brewers employ in the manufacture of beer, and which always affect the quality of their yeast, I am confident that domestic yeast can be made of a far superior quality. However light and good in other respects that bread may be which is made with brewers yeast, I have rarely if ever seen any in which I could not at once detect the disagreeable properties of the yeast.

There are various ways of making domestic yeast. One of the simplest, and perhaps the best, is the following, which was communicated to me by one of the best bread-makers I ever saw:

"Put into one gallon of water a double handful of hops;—boil them fifteen or twenty minutes, then strain off the water while it is scalding hot;—stir in wheat flour or meal till it becomes a thick batter, so that it will hardly pour;—let it stand till it becomes about blood warm, then add a pint of good lively yeast, and stir it well; and then let it stand in a place where it will be kept at a temperature of about 70° F. till it becomes perfectly light, whether more or less time is required; and then it is fit for use;—or if it is desired to keep a portion of it, let it stand several hours and become cool;

and then put it into a clean jug and cork it tight, and place it in the cellar where it will keep cool; and it may be preserved good, ten or twelve days, and even longer."

Another way by which yeast when thus made may be preserved much longer, and perhaps more conveniently, is, to take it when it has become perfectly light, and stir in good Indian meal until it becomes a hard dough: then take this dough and make it into small thin cakes, and dry them perfectly, without baking or cooking them at all. These cakes, if kept perfectly dry, will be good for several weeks and even months.

When yeast is needed, take some of these cakes (more or less according to the quantity of bread desired) and break them fine and dissolve them in warm water, and then stir in some wheat flour till a batter is formed, which should be kept at a temperature of about 60° F. till the yeast becomes light and lively, and fitted for making bread.

Others, in making this yeast, originally put into the water with the hops, a double handful of good clean wheat bran, and boil them up together and strain off the water as above described: others again, boil up a quantity of wheat bran without the hops, and make their yeast in all other respects as above described.

The milk yeast is greatly preferred by many; and when it is well managed, it certainly makes very handsome bread. The way of making it is simple. Take a quart of milk fresh from the cow, (more or less according to the quantity of bread desired,)—a little salt is generally added, and some add about half a pint of water blood warm, but this is not essential;—then stir wheat flour or meal into the milk till it forms a moderately thick batter; and then cover it over, and place it where it will remain at a temperature of from 60° to 70° F. till it becomes perfectly light. It should then be used immediately: and let it be remembered that dough made with this yeast will sour sooner than that made with other yeast; and also that the bread after it is baked will become extremely dry and *crumbly* much sooner than bread made with other yeast. Yet this bread, when a day old, is exceedingly light and beautiful: albeit some dislike the animal smell and taste which it derives from the milk.

In all these preparations of yeast and dough, it should ever be recollected that "the process of fermentation cannot go on when the temperature is below 30° F., that it proceeds quite slowly at 50°, moderately at 60°, rapidly at 70°, and very rapidly at 80°."

If, therefore, it is desired to have the yeast or dough stand several hours before it is used or baked, it should be kept at a temperature of about 50°. But in the ordinary way of making bread, a temperature varying from 60° to 70°, or about summer heat, is perhaps as near right as it can well be made.

Prof. Thomson gives the following directions for making yeast in large quantities:—"Add ten pounds of flour to two gallons of boiling water;—stir it well into a paste, let this mixture stand for seven hours, and then add about a quart of good yeast. In about six or eight hours, this mixture, if kept in a warm place, will have fermented and produced as much yeast as will make 120 quartern loaves" (of 4 lbs. each.)

A much smaller quantity can be made by observing due proportions of the ingredients.

To raise bread in a very short time without yeast, Prof. Thomson gives the following recipe:

"Dissolve in water 2 ounces, 5 drams and 45 grains of common crystallized carbonate of soda, and mix the solution well with your dough, and then add 7 ounces, 2 drams and 22 grains of muriatic acid of the specific gravity of 1,121, and knead it as rapidly as possible with your dough;—it will rise immediately—fully as much, if not more than dough mixed with yeast—and when baked, will be a very light and excellent bread." Smaller quantities would be required for small batches of bread.

A tea-spoonful or more (according to the quantity of dough or batter) of super-carbonate of soda dissolved in water, and flour stirred in till it becomes a batter, and then an equal quantity of tartaric acid dissolved and stirred in thoroughly, will in a few minutes make very light batter for griddle or pancakes; or if it be mixed into a thick dough, it will make light bread.

Good lively yeast, however, makes better bread than these alkalies and acids: howbeit these are very convenient in emergencies, when bread or cakes must be prepared in a very short time; or when the yeast has proved inefficient.

We see then that wheat meal consists of certain proportions of starch, gluten, sugar, bran, &c.; and that in making loaf bread, we add yeast or leaven, in order to produce that kind of fermentation peculiar to saccharine matter or sugar, which is called vinous, and by which the gas or air is formed that raises the dough. But the sugar is an incorporate part of every particle of the meal, and is therefore equally diffused throughout the whole mass; and hence if we would make the very best loaf bread, the fermentive principle or yeast must also be equally diffused throughout the whole mass, so that a suitable portion of yeast will be brought to act at the same time on every particle of saccharine matter in the mass.

But let us endeavor to understand this process of fermentation. To speak in the language of chemistry, sugar is composed of certain proportions of carbon, oxygen and hydrogen. The yeast, acting on the sugar, overcomes those affinities by which these substances are held in the constitutional arrangement of sugar, and the process of decay or decomposition of the sugar takes place, which is called vinous fermentation. By this process of decay, two other forms of matter are produced, of an essentially different nature from each other and from the sugar. One of them is called carbonic acid gas or air, being formed by a chemical combination of certain proportions of carbon and oxygen. The other is known by the name of alcohol, and consists of a chemical combination of certain proportions of carbon, oxygen, and hydrogen. Carbonic acid gas is also produced by animal respiration or breathing, by the combustion of wood, coal, &c. &c. and in other ways of nature and of art: but neither in nature nor in art is there any known way by which alcohol can be produced, except by that process of the decay or destruction of sugar called vinous fermentation.

The carbonic acid gas, produced in the manner I have stated, is the air which inflates or puffs up and swells out the bread, when there is sufficient gluten or other cohesive matter in the dough to prevent its escape.

If the dough be permitted to stand too long in a warm place, the fermentation, having destroyed most or all of the sugar, will begin to act on the starch and mucilage, and destroy their nature, and produce vinegar; and therefore this stage of it is called the acetous fermentation: and if it still be permitted to go on, it will next commence its work of destruction on the gluten; and this is called the putrefactive fermentation, because it in many respects resembles the putrefaction of animal matter.

The vinous fermentation, therefore, by which the dough is raised and made light, may be carried to all necessary extent, and still be limited in its action to the saccharine matter or sugar—leaving the starch and gluten, and other properties of the meal, uninjured; and this is the point at which the fermentation should be arrested by the heat that bakes the dough. If it be permitted to go beyond the sugar, and act on the mucilage and starch, and produce acidity, the excellence of the bread is in some degree irreparably destroyed. The acid may be neutralized by pearlash or soda, so that the bread shall not be sour; but still, something of the natural flavor of the bread is gone, and it is not possible by any earthly means to restore it; and this injury will always be in proportion to the extent to which the process of the acetous fermentation is permitted to go in destroying the nature of the starch, and the bread will be proportionably destitute of that natural sweetness and delicious richness essential to good bread. Yet it is almost universally true, both in public and domestic bread-making, that the acetous fermentation is allowed to take place; and saleratus, or soda, or some other chemical agent is employed to neutralize the acid. By this means we may have bread free from acidity, it is true, but it is also destitute of the best and most delicious properties of good bread; and generally, by the time it is twenty-four hours old—and this is particularly true of bakers' bread—it is as dry and tasteless and unsavory as if it were made of plaster of Paris.

Many bread-makers mix their saleratus or soda with their yeast, or introduce it when they mix their dough, so that if the acetous fermentation does take place, the acid is neutralized by the alkali, and therefore, not being perceived, it is supposed never to have existed, and the bread is called sweet and good; especially if a small quantity of molasses be employed in making the dough. Others far more wisely withhold their alkali till the dough is raised enough to mould into the loaf, and then if it is found to be in any degree acid, a solution of saleratus or soda is worked into it, so as just to neutralize the acid, and no more. This is infinitely better that no have sour bread, which, after all, is almost everywhere met with; yet the very best bread that can be made in this way is only second best. Happy are they who can make good light and sweet bread, without the use of molasses—without suffering the least degree of acetous fermentation to take place, and without employing saleratus, soda, or any other kind of alkali.

The third or putrefactive stage of fermentation rarely takes place in domestic bread-making; but it is by no means uncommon in public bakeries. Indeed it is thought necessary in the manufacture of certain kinds of crackers, in order to make them split open, and render them brittle, and cause them readily to become soft when dipped into water. But dyspepsia crackers, and all other kinds of bread made in this way are, to say the least of them, miserable stuff. For besides the fact that all the best qualities of the flour or meal have been destroyed by fermentation, the great quantity of alkali employed in neutralizing the acid, is necessarily injurious to the digestive organs.

PREPARATION OF BREAD.

Mixing. Much kneading necessary. Rising, or fermentation. Use of alkalies, saleratus and soda. Baking. Ovens. Alcohol in bread. Preservation of bread.

Now, then, the business of the bread-maker is, to take the wheat meal, prepared in the manner I have stated, and with all the properties I have described, and convert it into good, light, sweet, well-baked bread, with the least possible change in those properties; so that the bread, when done, will present to the senses of smell and taste, all the delicious flavor and delicate sweetness which pure organs perceive in the meal of good new wheat, just taken from the ear and ground, or chewed without grinding; and it should be so baked that it will, as a general statement, require and secure a full exercise of the teeth in mastication.

In order to do this, as we have seen, it is necessary, in the first place, that the wheat should be of the best kind, and well cleansed, and the meal properly prepared. In the next place, it is necessary that the yeast should be fresh, lively and sweet; and in the third place, it is necessary that the dough should be properly mixed, raised and baked.

Take then such a quantity of meal, in a perfectly clean and sweet bread trough, as is necessary for the quantity of bread desired, and having made a hollow in the centre, turn in as much yeast as a judgment matured by sound experience shall deem requisite; then add such a quantity of water, milk and water, or clear milk, as is necessary to form the meal into a dough of proper consistency. Some prefer bread mixed with water alone; others prefer that which is mixed with milk and water; and others think that bread mixed with good milk is much richer and better; while others dislike the animal odor and taste of bread mixed with milk. Perhaps the very best and most wholesome bread is that which is mixed with pure soft water, when such bread is made perfect. But whether water, milk and water, or milk alone is employed, it should be used at a temperature of about blood heat.

Here let it be understood, that the starch of the meal is of such a nature that, by a delicate process peculiar to itself, it becomes changed into sugar or saccharine matter; and when the fluid used in mixing the dough is of a proper temperature, and the dough is properly mixed and kneaded, this process, to some small extent, takes place, and a small portion of the starch is actually converted into sugar, and thereby increases the sweetness of the bread. Let it also be recollected here, that the saccharine matter on which the yeast is to act, is equally diffused throughout the whole mass of the meal; and therefore if the yeast be not properly diffused throughout the whole mass, but is unequally distributed, so that an undue quantity of it remains in one part, while other parts receive little or none, then the fermentation will go on very rapidly in some parts of the mass, and soon run into the acetous state, while in other parts it will proceed very slowly or not at all; and consequently large cavities will be formed in some parts of the dough, while other parts of it will remain as compact and heavy as when first mixed, and sometimes even more so. I need not say that such dough cannot be made into good bread; yet it is probably true, that more than nine tenths of the bread consumed in this country is more or less of this character. Nor, after what I have said, should it seem necessary for me to remark, that good bread cannot be made by merely stirring the meal, and yeast, and water or milk together into a thin dough or sponge, and suffering it to ferment with little or no working or kneading. Bread made in this manner, if it is not full of cavities large enough for a mouse to burrow in, surrounded by parts as solid as lead, is almost invariably full of cells of the size of large peas and grapes; and the substance of the bread has a shining, glutinous appearance; and if the bread is not sour, it is because pearlash or some other kind of alkali has been used to destroy the acid.

The very appearance of such bread is forbidding, and shows, at a glance, that it has not been properly mixed—that the yeast has acted unequally on different portions of the meal, and that the fermentation has not been of the right kind.

But if the yeast be so diffused throughout the whole mass, as that a suitable portion of it will act on each and every particle of the saccharine matter at the same time, and if the dough be of such a consistency and temperature as not to admit of too rapid a fermentation, then each minute portion of saccharine matter throughout the whole mass will, in the process of fermentation, produce its little volume of air, which will form its little cell, about the size of a pin's head, and smaller; and this will take place so nearly at the same time, in every part of the dough, that the whole will be raised and made as light as a sponge, before the acetous fermentation takes place in any part. And then if it be properly moulded and baked, it will make the most beautiful and delicious bread—perfectly light and sweet, without the use of any alkali, and with all the gluten and nearly all the starch of the meal remaining unchanged by fermentation.

Proper materials, proper care, a due amount of labor, a suitable length of time, and proper temperature, are all, therefore, necessary to the making of good bread.

With your meal, and yeast, and water or milk brought together before you, then, proceed in the light of the instruction you have now received, to mix your dough; and remember that the more thoroughly you knead it, the more equally you diffuse the yeast throughout the whole mass, and bring it to act on every particle of the saccharine matter at the same time, and the whiter, lighter, and more delicious you make your bread.

Who that can look back thirty or forty years to those blessed days of New England's prosperity and happiness, when our good mothers used to make the family bread, but can well remember how long and how patiently those excellent matrons stood over their bread troughs, kneading and moulding their dough? and who with such recollections cannot also well remember the delicious bread that these mothers used invariably to set before them? There was a natural sweetness and richness in it which made it always desirable; and which we cannot now vividly recollect, without feeling a strong desire to partake again of such bread as our mothers made for us in the days of our childhood.

Let it be borne in mind, then, that without a very thorough kneading of the dough, there can be no just ground of confidence that the bread will be good. "It should be kneaded," says one of much experience in this matter, "till it becomes flaky." Indeed I am confident that our loaf bread would be greatly improved in all its qualities, if the dough were for a considerable time subjected to the operations of the machine which the bakers call the break, used in making crackers and sea-bread.

The wheat meal, and especially if it is ground coarsely, swells considerably in the dough, and therefore the dough should not, at first, be made quite so stiff, as that made of superfine flour; and when it is raised, if it is found too soft to mould well, let a little more meal be added.

When the dough has been properly mixed and thoroughly kneaded, cover it over with a clean napkin or towel, and a light woollen blanket kept for the purpose, and place the bread trough where the temperature will be kept at about 60° F., or about summer heat, and there let it remain till the dough becomes light. But as it is impossible to regulate the quantity and quality of your yeast, the moisture and temperature of your dough, and several other conditions and circumstances, so as to secure at all times precisely the same results in the same time, it is therefore necessary that careful attention should be given that the proper moment should be seized to work over and mould the dough into the loaf, and get it into the oven, just at the time when it is as light as it can be made by the vinous fermentation, and before the acetous fermentation commences.

If, however, by any means there should unfortunately be a little acidity in the dough, take a small quantity of saleratus, or, what is better, carbonate of soda, and dissolve it in some warm water, and carefully work in just enough to neutralize the acid. The best bread-makers are so exceedingly careful on this point, that they dip their fingers into the solution of saleratus or soda, and thrust them into the dough in every part, as they work it over, so as to be sure that they get in just enough to neutralize the acid, and not a particle more.

I must here repeat, that they who would have the very best of bread, must always consider it a cause of regret, that there should be any necessity to use alkali; because the acetous fermentation cannot in any degree take place, without commensurately and irremediably impairing the quality of the bread. And here it should be remarked, that dough made of wheat meal will take on the acetous fermentation, or become sour, sooner than that made of fine flour. This is probably owing principally to the mucilage contained in the bran, which runs into the acetous fermentation sooner than starch.

While the dough is rising, preparations should be made for baking it. Some bake their bread in a brick oven, some in a stove, some in a reflector, and some in a baking kettle. In all these ways very good bread may be baked; but the baking kettle is decidedly the most objectionable. Probably there is no better and more certain way of baking bread well than in the use of the brick oven. Good bread-makers, accustomed to brick ovens, can always manage them with a very great degree of certainty; and as a general fact, bread is sweeter, baked in this way, than in any other. Yet, when it is well baked in tin reflectors, it is certainly very fine; and so it is also when well baked in iron stoves. But the baking of bread requires almost as much care and judgment as any part of the process of bread-making. If the oven is too hot, the bread will burn on the outside before it is done in the centre; if it is too cold, the bread will be heavy, raw and sour. If the heat is much greater from below than from above, the bottom of the loaf will burn before the top is done: or if the heat is much greater from above than from below, the top of the loaf will burn before the bottom is done.

All these points therefore must be carefully attended to; and no small excuse ought to be considered a satisfactory apology for sour, heavy, raw or burnt bread; for it is hardly possible to conceive of an absolute necessity for such results; and the cases are extremely rare in which they are not the offspring of downright and culpable carelessness.

The best bread-makers I have ever known, watch over their bread troughs while their dough is rising, and over their ovens while it is baking, with about as much care and attention as a mother watches over the cradle of her sick child.

Dough made of wheat meal requires a hotter oven than that made of fine flour; and it needs to remain in the oven longer. Indeed, it is a general fault of bread of every description, made in this country, that it is not sufficiently baked. Multitudes eat their bread hot and smoking from the oven in a half-cooked state; and very few seem to think there is any impropriety in doing so. But they who would have their bread good, not only a few hours after it comes from the oven, but as long as it can be kept, must see that it is thoroughly baked.

I have said that the process of vinous fermentation converts a portion of the saccharine matter of the meal into carbonic acid gas or air, by which means the dough is raised and made light; and that the same process converts a portion of the saccharine matter into alcohol. The alcohol thus generated is mostly if not entirely driven off by the heat of the oven when the dough is baking;—and in modern times, ovens have been so constructed in England, as to serve the double purpose of ovens and stills; so that while the bread is baking, the alcohol is distilled off and condensed, and saved for the various uses of arts and manufacture.

The question has, however, been frequently started, whether a portion of the alcohol thus generated, is not contained in the bread when it comes from the oven.

This question cannot be answered with entire certainty; but there are some facts in relation to it of considerable importance.

It is perfectly certain that if two portions of wheat meal or flour be taken from the same barrel or sack, and one portion be made into unleavened bread, and the other portion be made into the very best fermented or raised bread, and both be eaten as soon as they are baked, the fermented bread will digest with more difficulty, and oppress and disturb the stomach more than the unleavened bread will. Indeed it is well known and very generally understood, that few of the articles which compose the food of man in civic life, are so trying to the human stomach, and so powerful causes of dyspepsia, as fresh-baked raised bread.

It is now well known also that alcohol wholly resists the action of the solvent fluid of the stomach, and is entirely indigestible; and always retards the digestion of those substances which contain it. How far all this may be true of carbonic acid gas, is not yet ascertained; but it is difficult to account for the difference between leavened and unleavened bread, as above stated, without supposing that the alcohol or carbonic acid gas, or both of them, are in some degree concerned in rendering the leavened bread, when newly baked, peculiarly oppressive and injurious to the stomach.

This, be it remembered, is purely a conjecture of my own; and I am not entirely certain that it is correct; but I see no other way of meeting the difficulty.

Be it as it may, however, it is very certain that when the bread has been drawn from the oven, and permitted to stand in a proper place twenty-four hours, either by evaporation or some other means, it becomes perfectly matured, and so changed in character, that it is, if properly made, one of the most wholesome articles entering into the diet of man; and at that age, there is not the slightest reason to believe that a particle of alcohol remains in the bread.

When therefore the bread is thoroughly baked, let it be taken from the oven and placed on a perfectly clean and sweet shelf, in a perfectly clean and well ventilated pantry. Do not, as you value the character of your bread, put it into a pantry where you set away dishes of cold meat, cold potatoes, and other vegetables, and keep your butter, cheese and various other table provisions—in a pantry which perhaps is seldom thoroughly cleansed with hot water and soap, and where the pure air of heaven seldom if ever has a free circulation. The quality of your bread should be of too much importance to allow of such reprehensible carelessness, not to say sluttishness. And if you will have your bread such as every one ought to desire to have it, you must pay the strictest attention to the cleanliness and sweetness of the place where you keep it.

If in baking, the outer crust should become a little too dry and crispy, you can easily remedy this by throwing a clean bread or table cloth over it for a short time when it first comes from the oven; but if this is not necessary, let the bread stand on an airy shelf, till it becomes perfectly cool, and when it is twenty-four hours old, it is fit for use; and if it is in all respects properly made, and properly kept, it will continue to be sweet and delicious bread for two or even three weeks, except perhaps in very hot and sultry weather.

When we have acquired the art of making such bread as I have described, in the very best manner, then have we carried the art of cooking to the very height of perfection; for it is not only true, that there is no other artificially prepared article in human diet of so much importance as bread, but it is also true that there is no other preparation in the whole round of cooking, which requires so much care, and attention, and experience, and skill, and wisdom.

WHO SHOULD MAKE BREAD.

Making bread by rule. Bakers. Domestics. Sour bread. An anecdote. Mrs. Van Winkle. Bad bread need not be made. How cake is made. Bread-making a drudgery. Excellent example of a mother. Eating bad bread. Importance of having good bread.

Who then shall make our bread? For after all that science in its utmost accuracy can do, in ascertaining principles and in laying down rules, there is little certainty that any one, who undertakes to make bread merely by rule, will be anything like uniformly successful. We may make a batch of bread according to certain rules, and it may prove excellent; and then we may make another batch according to the same rules, which may be very poor. For if we follow our rules ever so closely, there may be some slight differences in the quality or condition of the meal or the yeast, or something else, which will materially alter the character of the bread, if we do not exercise a proper care and judgment, and vary our operations according as the particular circumstances of the case may require.

Correct rules are certainly very valuable; but they can only serve as general way-marks, in the art of bread-making. Uniform success can only be secured by the exercise of that mature judgment which is always able to dictate those extemporaneous measures which every exigency and circumstance may require; and such a judgment can only result from a care and attention and experience which are the offspring of that moral sensibility which duly appreciates the importance of the quality of bread, in relation to the happiness and welfare of those that consume it.

But are we to look for such a sensibility in public bakers? Can we expect that they will feel so lively and so strong an interest for our enjoyment and for our physical and intellectual and moral well-being, that they will exercise all that care and attention and patience, and watch with that untiring vigilance and solicitude in all the progress of their operations, which are indispensably necessary in order to secure us the best of bread?

Or can we reasonably expect to find these qualifications in domestics—in those who serve us for hire? Many a female domestic, it is true, can make much better bread than her mistress can. Many a female domestic has an honest and sincere desire to do her duty faithfully; but can she be actuated by those sensibilities and affections which alone can secure that careful attention, that soundness of judgment, that accuracy of operation, without which the best of bread cannot uniformly, if ever, be produced?

No;—it is the wife, the mother only—she who loves her husband and her children as woman ought to love, and who rightly perceives the relations between the dietetic habits and physical and moral condition of her loved ones, and justly appreciates the importance of good bread to their physical and moral welfare—she alone it is, who will be ever inspired by that cordial and unremitting affection and solicitude which will excite the vigilance, secure the attention, and prompt the action requisite to success, and essential to the attainment of that maturity of judgment and skilfulness of operation, which are the indispensable attributes of a perfect bread-maker. And could wives and mothers fully comprehend the importance of good bread in relation to all the bodily and intellectual and moral interests of their husbands and children, and in relation to the domestic and social and civil welfare of mankind, and to their religious prosperity, both for time and eternity, they would estimate the art and duty of bread-making far, very far more highly than they now do. They would then realize that, as no one can feel so deep and delicate an interest for their husbands' and children's happiness as they do, so no one can be so proper a person to prepare for them that portion of their aliment, which requires a degree of care and attention that can only spring from the lively affections and solicitude of a wife and mother.

But it is a common thing to hear women say—"We cannot always have good bread, if we take ever so much pains;—it will sometimes be heavy, and sometimes be sour, and sometimes badly baked, in spite of all our care."

It may be true that such things will sometimes happen, even with the best of care;—but I believe that there is almost infinitely more poor bread than there is any good excuse for. The truth is, the quality of bread is a matter of too little consideration; and therefore too little care is given to the making of it. Moreover, the sense of taste is so easily vitiated, that we can very easily become reconciled to the most offensive gustatory qualities, and even learn to love them; and it is a very common thing to find families so accustomed to sour bread, that they have no perception of its acid quality.

"It is very strange," said a lady to me one day at her dinner table, "that some folks always have sour bread, and never know it." She then went on to name a number of families in the circle of her acquaintance, who, she said, invariably had sour bread upon their tables when she visited them—"and they never," continued she, "seem to have the least consciousness that their bread is not perfectly sweet and good."

Yet this very lady, at the very moment she was thus addressing me, had sour bread upon her own table; and although I had for many months been very frequently at her table, I had never found any but sour bread upon it. Still she was wholly unconscious of the fact.

Difficult however as most women think it is, to have good bread always, yet there are some women who invariably have excellent bread. I have known such women. The wife of Thomans Van Winkle, Esq. of the beautiful valley of Booneton, New Jersey—peace to her ashes!—was deservedly celebrated throughout the whole circle of her acquaintance for her excellent bread. Few ever ate at her hospitable board once that did not desire to enjoy the privilege again. I know not how often it has been my good fortune to sit at her table; but the times have not been few; and though long past, and she who presided there has slept for years in her grave, yet the remembrance of those times and of those hospitalities, awakens in my bosom a deep and fervent sentiment of gratitude while I write.

Never at the table of Mrs. Van Winkle did I eat poor bread;—and of my numerous acquaintances who had sat at her table, I never heard one say he had eaten poor bread there. Her bread was invariably good. Nay, it was of such a quality that it was impossible for any one to eat of it, and not be conscious that he was partaking of bread of extraordinary excellence.

Mrs. Van Winkle, said I to her one day, while I was feasting on her delicious bread, tell me truly, is there either a miracle or mystery in this matter of bread-making, by which you are enabled to have such excellent bread upon your table at all times, while I rarely ever find bread equally good at any other table, and at ninety-nine tables in a hundred, I almost invariably find poor bread? Is it necessarily so? Is it not possible for people by any means to have good bread uniformly?

"There is no necessity for having poor bread at any time, if those who make it will give proper care and attention to their business," replied Mrs. Van Winkle, confidently. "The truth is," continued she, "most people attach very little importance to the quality of their bread; and therefore they give little care to the preparation of it. If every woman would see that her flour is sweet and good, that her yeast is fresh and lively, that her bread trough is kept perfectly clean and sweet, that her dough is properly mixed and thoroughly kneaded, and kept at a proper temperature, and at the proper time moulded into the loaf, and put into the oven, which has been properly heated, and there properly baked, then good bread would be as common as poor bread now is. But while there is such perfect carelessness and negligence about the matter, it is not surprising that bread should be generally poor."

Mrs. Van Winkle was undoubtedly correct. If anything like the care were given to bread-making that its real importance demands, a loaf of poor bread would rarely be met with. Indeed, if the same degree of care were given to bread-making, that is devoted to the making of cakes and pastry, we should far more generally be blessed with good bread.

Who does not know, that as soon as girls are old enough to go into company and to give parties, they begin to notice with great interest the qualities of the different kinds of cake and pastry which they meet with; and whenever they find anything very nice, they are exceedingly curious to learn precisely how it was made. And lest memory should be treacherous, they will carefully write down the exact rules for mixing and cooking it;—"so many pounds of flour, so many pounds of butter, so many pounds of sugar, so many eggs, and spice to your taste—the eggs to be beaten so and so, the whole mixed so and so, and baked so many minutes," &c. &c. And thus with great care and industry they collect and write down, in a book which they keep for the purpose, all the recipes they can get hold of, for making every kind of cake and pastry used in society. And when they are preparing for company, they rarely if ever order Dinah or any other domestic to make their nice cake. They do not regard it as a menial office, but as a highly genteel employment; and their great desire to have their cake and pastry as good as it can be made, prompts them to undertake the manufacture of it themselves. And during this operation, the scales, the measures, the clock or watch, all are brought into requisition; the Recipe Book is placed upon the table before them, and carefully consulted; and everything is done with the utmost precision, and exactitude, and vigilance. And if the young lady feels any misgiving as to her own judgment, or taste, or experience, she earnestly inquires of Ma, or some one else who she thinks is capable of giving her advice in so important a matter.

If in the midst of this employment some one knocks or rings at the door, and a young gentleman is announced, she is not at all embarrassed, but perhaps hastens to the parlor with her delicate hands covered with dough, and with an air of complacency and self-satisfaction, says—"Good morning, Frank—how do you do? I am just engaged in making some cake—I hope you will excuse me for a few moments."

All this shows that she regards the quality of her cake as of very great importance, and considers it not only perfectly respectable but highly *genteel*, for a young lady to be employed in making cake. But in regard to bread and bread-making, everything is very different; there is none of this early curiosity to learn how to make good bread. Young ladies do not on every occasion when they find excellent bread, carefully and minutely inquire how it was made, baked, &c., and write down the recipe;—but when a batch of bread is to be made for the family, they either leave it for Mother or some domestic to make, or go about it themselves as some irksome and disreputable piece of drudgery; and consequently they turn the task off their hands with as much despatch and as little trouble as possible. If all things happen to be as they should be, it is well; if not, they must answer for the present. If the yeast happens to be lively and sweet, very lucky. If otherwise, still it must be used. If the dough rises well and is got into the oven before it becomes sour, very fortunate; if not, why, "nobody can avoid mistakes—and bread will sometimes be poor in spite of the greatest care;"—and if a batch of miserable bread is the result of such an operation, then all that remains to be done is to eat it up as soon as possible, and hope for better the next time.

If Frank or Charles or Edward should call while the young lady is engaged in making bread, she is perhaps quite disconcerted, and would not for the world have him know what she is doing;—she sends word to him, either that she is out, or that she is particularly engaged, and begs he will excuse her;—or if by any means she happens unexpectedly to be caught at her employment, she is greatly embarrassed, and makes the best apology she can for being engaged in such menial services.

As a matter of course, while such are the views and feelings entertained on this subject, and while such is the manner in which this duty is performed, it will ever be a mere accident if good bread is made; and a mere accident if such girls ever become good bread-makers when they are wives and mothers.

But if parents, and especially mothers, could view this matter in its true light, how differently would they educate their children. They would then feel that, grateful as it is to a mother's heart to see her daughters highly refined and elegantly accomplished, and able to "make the instrument discourse most eloquent music," and to transfer living nature, with all its truth and beauty and sublimity, to the canvass, still the art of bread-making, when considered in all its relations and intimate connections with human health, and prosperity, and virtue, and happiness, and with reference to the natural responsibilities and duties of woman, is actually one of the highest and noblest accomplishments that can adorn the female character. And then, too, would they consider it of exceedingly great importance, that their daughters should possess this accomplishment, even though they may never be in circumstances which will require the exercise of it.

Some eight or nine years since, I spent several months in the delightful village of Belvidere, on the banks of the Delaware, in Pennsylvania. While there, I enjoyed for a number of weeks the kind hospitality of S— S—, Esq., a lawyer, and a gentleman of great moral excellence. Mrs. S. was born and brought up, I believe, in Philadelphia. Her father was a man of wealth, and she was the only daughter, and—almost as a matter of course—was indulged in all that she desired. But there were so many of the elements of a good wife and mother in her natural composition, that as soon as she entered into those interesting and important relations, she began to devote herself to the duties of them with a sincerity and conscientiousness which could not fail of success. Surrounded as she was, with wealth, and every comfort and convenience of life, and all of its luxuries that she desired, still she was industrious in her habits, and vigilantly attentive to all the concerns of her household. She usually kept three female domestics, who, by her kind maternal deportment towards them, were warmly attached to her. She had no difficulty in procuring nor in keeping help, because she always treated them in such a manner that they loved to stay with her; and she took much pains to qualify them for the proper discharge of their duties. They evidently loved her, and were sincerely desirous of performing all their services in such a manner as would be pleasing to her. Yet with all these advantages to justify her leaving such a duty to her domestics, Mrs. S. invariably made the family bread with her own hands. Regularly as the baking day came, she went into her kitchen and took her stand beside the bread trough, and mixed and kneaded the dough, and put it in its proper place for rising, and, in due time, moulded it into the loaf and baked it.

Do you always make your bread, madam? I inquired one day, as she returned from the performance of that task. "Invariably," she replied: "that is a duty I trust no other person to do for me."

But cannot your domestics make good bread? I asked. "I have excellent domestics," answered Mrs. S., "and they can, perhaps, make as good bread as I can; for they have been with me several years, and I have taken pains to learn them how to do my work; and they are exceedingly faithful and affectionate, and are always willing to do all they can to please me; but they cannot feel for my husband and my children as I do, and therefore they cannot feel that interest which I do, in always having such bread as my husband and my children will love and enjoy. Besides, if it were certain their care and vigilance and success in bread-making would be always equal to mine, yet it is wholly uncertain how long they will remain with me. Various circumstances may take place, which may cause them to leave me, and bring me into dependence upon those who know not how to make good bread; and therefore I choose to keep my own hand in. But, apart from all other considerations, there is a pleasure resulting from the performance of this duty, which richly rewards me for all the labor of it. When my bread is made and brought upon the table, and I see my husband and children eat it and enjoy it, and hear them speak of its excellence, it affords me much satisfaction, and I am glad to know that I have contributed so much to their health and happiness; for, while my bread is so good that they prefer it to anything else upon the table, there is little danger of their indulging, to any injurious extent, in those articles of food which are less favorable to their health."

I need not say that this lady invariably had excellent bread upon her table. But instances of this kind are, I regret to say, extremely rare, even in christian communities; and therefore when such cases are known, they ought to be held up as most noble examples of female virtue, and receive such high commendations as their intrinsic merit deserves, and such as will be calculated to beget in the minds of others an exalted sense of the dignity and importance of such duties, and prompt every wife and mother to the intelligent and affectionate performance of them.

For it should ever be remembered that, though our children, while they depend on us for protection, are also properly the subjects of our government, yet as soon as they are capable of appreciating our authority and our influence, they are, like ourselves, moral agents, and ought, in all respects, to be governed and nurtured as such; and therefore it is not enough that we can give them such bread as we think best for them, and *compel* them to eat it; but the grand point at which the mother should always aim, in this matter, is, to place before her children such bread as is the very best for them, and at the same time, to make it the most agreeable to them, and thereby make their duty and their enjoyment perfectly coincide.

Let no one therefore say she cannot always have good bread, until she can truly affirm that she has fairly made the experiment; that she has, in view of all its relations and bearings, accurately estimated the importance of the quality of her bread in regard to the welfare of her household, and, with a proper sense of her responsibilities as a wife and mother, has *at all times* felt that interest and exercised that care and attention which so important a duty demands, and without which it must ever be a mere accident whether her bread is good or bad.

They that will have good bread, not only for a single time, but uniformly, must make the quality of their bread of sufficient importance, in their estimation and feelings, to secure the requisite attention to the means by which alone such an end can be made certain. They must not suffer themselves, through carelessness, to get entirely out of bread unexpectedly, and thus be obliged, without due preparation, to make up a batch of such materials as they may happen to have at hand, and bake it in haste, and hurry it to the table. But they must exercise providence and foresight: they must know, beforehand, when their supply of bread will probably be out, and when they will need to make another batch; and they must see beforehand that measures are taken to secure a proper supply of all the requisite materials—see that they are furnished with good meal or flour; and they must be sure to have the best of yeast or leaven, when they need it —and when the time comes for them to make their bread, if by any means the yeast should not be good, let them throw it away and make good, before they proceed to make their bread; for it is infinitely better that the family should even do without bread one day, and eat roasted potatoes, than that they should eat poor bread three or four days; and if, from any cause, the bread should be poor, it is incomparably better to throw it away, than to set it upon the table, to disgust the whole family with bread, and drive them to make most of their meal on something else.

If a lady can ever find a good excuse for having poor bread, she certainly can find none, except perhaps extreme poverty, for setting her poor bread on the table the second time. Yet, too generally, women seem to think that, as a matter of course, if they, by carelessness or any other means, have been so unlucky as to make a batch of poor bread, their family and friends must share their misfortune, and help them eat it up; and, by this means, many a child has had its health seriously impaired, and its constitution injured, and perhaps its moral character ruined—by being driven, in early life, into pernicious dietetic habits.

It was observed many years ago, by one of the most eminent and extensive practitioners in New England, that, during a practice of medicine for thirty years, he had always remarked that, in those families where the children were most afflicted with worms, he invariably found poor bread; and that, as a general fact, the converse of this was true; that is, in those families where they uniformly had heavy, sour, ill-baked bread, he generally found that the children were afflicted with worms.

A careful and extensive observation for a few years, would convince every intelligent mind that there is a far more intimate relation between the quality of the bread and the moral character of a family, than is generally supposed.

"Keep that man at least ten paces from you, who eats no bread with his dinner," said Lavater, in his "Aphorisms on Man." This notion appears to be purely whimsical at first glance; but Lavater was a shrewd observer, and seldom erred in the moral inferences which he drew from the voluntary habits of mankind; and depend upon it, a serious contemplation of this apparent whim, discloses a deeper philosophy than is at first perceived upon the surface.

Whatever may be the cause which turns our children and ourselves away from the dish of bread, and establishes an habitual disregard for it, the effect, though not perhaps in every individual instance, yet, as a general fact, is certainly, in some degree, unfavorable to the physical, and intellectual, and moral, and religious, and social, and civil and political interests of man.

Of all the artificially prepared articles of food which come upon our table, therefore, bread should be that one which, as a general fact, is uniformly preferred by our children and our household,—that one, the absence of which they would notice soonest, and feel the most,—that one which—however they may enjoy for a time the little varieties set before them—they would be most unwilling to dispense with—and which, if they were driven to the necessity, they would prefer to any other dish, as a single article of subsistence.

To effect this state of things, it is obvious that the quality of the bread must be uniformly excellent; and to secure this, I say again, there must be a judgment, an experience, a skill, a care, a vigilance, which can only spring from the sincere affections of a devoted wife and mother, who accurately perceives and duly appreciates the importance of these things, and, in the lively exercise of a pure and delicate moral sense, feels deeply her responsibilities, and is prompted to the performance of her duties.

Would to God that this were all true of every wife and mother in our country—in the world!—that the true relations, and interests, and responsibilities of life were understood and felt by every human being, and all the duties of life properly and faithfully performed!

www.ingramcontent.com/pod-product-compliance
Lightning Source LLC
Chambersburg PA
CBHW081732100526
44591CB00016B/2593